NATURAL WAYS TO PREVENT HAIR LOSS

AND

TO REGROW HAIR

Dr Nyjon K Eccles

BSc MBBS MRCP PhD

NATURAL WAYS TO PREVENT HAIR LOSS AND TO REGROW HAIR

© El Roble Edition

All right reserved

El Roble Editions
U.S.A.

www.elroble.us

All rights reserved. No portion of this book may be reproduced, stored in a retrieval system, or transmitted in any form or by any means - electronic, mechanical, photocopy, recording, scanning, or other - except for a brief quotation in critical reviews or articles, without the prior written permission of the publisher.

Published in Spain 2024 05   First edition

ISBN: 979-832-202-2084

The book can be ordered directly at: order@www.elroble.us

Or on the website: elroble.us/regrowhair

Thank you and dedication

I dedicate this book to my wife Nina. It is because of her support and patience that I have been able to find the time to write this book. I am eternally grateful for her understanding despite her maverick husband; spending time in his cave seeking to at least solve some of the health challenges that face us.

Thanks also to all my clinic staff- especially Zuzana, my practice manager, who has been there in recent years to support the mad scientist in me and for her help drive our clinic, The Natural Doctor, to excellence.

I must also say thanks to Philippe Lange, who has helped in the preparation and publication of this book but also for his foresight as a business colleague and friend. We will together do some good.

About the author

Dr Nyjon Eccles BSc, MBBS, MRCP, PhD is one of the most respected Integrated Medicine physicians in the UK and has been at the forefront in the use of pioneering, innovative and ground breaking natural healthcare over the last decade.

He holds a raft of medical and academic qualifications, including the MBBS, and is a Member of the Royal College of Physicians (MRCP). He also holds a PhD in Pharmacology (London).

Over the years, Dr Eccles has built an enviable reputation as a champion for men and women looking for access to a wider range of treatment and prevention options in managing their health.

Practicing from a Central London clinic, The Natural Doctor, Dr Eccles specialises in Thermocheck® Breast Thermography, Natural Menopause treatment, including Natural Bioidentical Hormone Replacement, Better Ageing programs and Natural BioGroHair® Restoration (having developed a revolutionary effective formula which is International patent pending).

The Natural Doctor prevention is at the heart of everything Dr Eccles does. The aim is to strengthen the body against disease, illness and ageing in the most natural, non-invasive and safe ways possible and using pioneering treatments, many of which have been designed as a result of my years of experience in conventional and natural medical practice and pharmacology.

Table of Contents

About the author — 5

Physiological Mechanisms of Hair Loss in Men and Women — 9

Inflammation and Oxidative Stress: Their Role in Hair Loss — 13

Oxidative Stress and Hair Loss — 15

The Significance of Circulation in Hair Loss — 19

Nutrient Deficiency and Hair Loss: Scientific Evidence and Corrective Supplemental Doses — 23

Vitamin D Deficiency and Hair Loss: Unveiling the Evidence — 27

Genetics and Hair Loss: Its Role in Men and Women — 31

The Role of Estrogen and Progesterone in Hair Growth and Quality: Relation to menopause-associated hair fall — 37

Minoxidil and Propecia for Male Pattern Hair Loss: Efficacy and Side Effects — 43

Side Effects of Propecia in Male Hair Loss Treatments: Current Legal Cases — 49

Lifestyle Factors and Hair Loss in Men and Women: Understanding the Connection — 53

Hair Transplantation: Considerations and Risks — 59

Essential Oils for Hair Loss: Exploring the Scientific Evidence — 65

The Development of BioGroHair®: The Need For a Safer and More Effective Non-Surgical Hair Restoration Program — 69

BioGroHair®: A novel innovation in hair restoration	73
MALE Testimonials	77
FEMALE Testimonials	81
Final Comments	82
How to get BioGroHair® with special offer?	85

Physiological Mechanisms of Hair Loss in Men and Women

Introduction

Hair loss, scientifically known as alopecia, is a common concern for both men and women. Understanding the physiological mechanisms underlying hair loss is crucial for developing effective prevention and treatment strategies. In this chapter, we will explore the known physiological mechanisms of hair loss in both genders, supported by scientific references.

1. *Androgenetic Alopecia (AGA)*

Androgenetic alopecia, commonly referred to as male pattern baldness in men and female pattern hair loss in women, is the most prevalent form of hair loss in both sexes. It is primarily driven by hormonal and genetic factors.

- In Men: In men, the hormone dihydrotestosterone (DHT), a derivative of testosterone, plays a pivotal role in AGA. DHT binds to specific receptors on hair follicles, initiating a miniaturization process[1]. This process results in the gradual reduction of hair follicle size, leading to shorter, finer hair and eventually hair loss.

- In Women: In women with AGA, the mechanisms are more complex. While DHT is still involved, hormonal imbalances, including elevated levels of androgens, contribute to hair thinning and loss[2]. Genetic predisposition also plays a role in determining susceptibility to AGA in women.

2. Telogen Effluvium

Telogen effluvium is a transient form of hair loss triggered by various physiological stressors. It occurs when a significant number of hair follicles simultaneously enter the resting (telogen) phase of the hair growth cycle.

- In Men and Women: Telogen effluvium can affect individuals of both genders. Common triggers include physical or emotional stress, illness, childbirth, medication changes, and extreme weight loss[3]. The stressor disrupts the normal hair growth cycle, leading to excessive shedding. Fortunately, this type of hair loss is usually reversible once the underlying cause is addressed.

3. Alopecia Areata

Alopecia areata is an autoimmune condition in which the immune system mistakenly attacks hair follicles.

- In Men and Women: Both men and women can develop alopecia areata, characterized by the sudden appearance of round, patchy areas of hair loss on the scalp or other parts of the body[4]. The exact cause of this autoimmune response remains unclear, but it likely involves genetic and environmental factors.

4. Traction Alopecia

Traction alopecia results from persistent tension or pulling on the hair, often due to tight hairstyles such as braids, ponytails, or extensions.

- In Men and Women: Traction alopecia can affect individuals of both sexes, but it is more commonly associated with certain hairstyling practices. The repeated mechanical stress on hair follicles can lead to inflammation and damage over time[5].

5. *Nutritional Deficiencies*

Inadequate nutrition can also contribute to hair loss.

- In Men and Women: Deficiencies in essential nutrients, such as iron, zinc, biotin, and certain vitamins (especially vitamin D), can affect the health of hair follicles and lead to hair loss[6][7].

Conclusion

Hair loss in both men and women involves a range of physiological mechanisms. Understanding these mechanisms is essential for identifying the underlying causes of hair loss and developing effective treatment strategies. It's important to remember that individual cases of hair loss can be unique, with multiple factors interacting to produce the observed hair loss pattern.

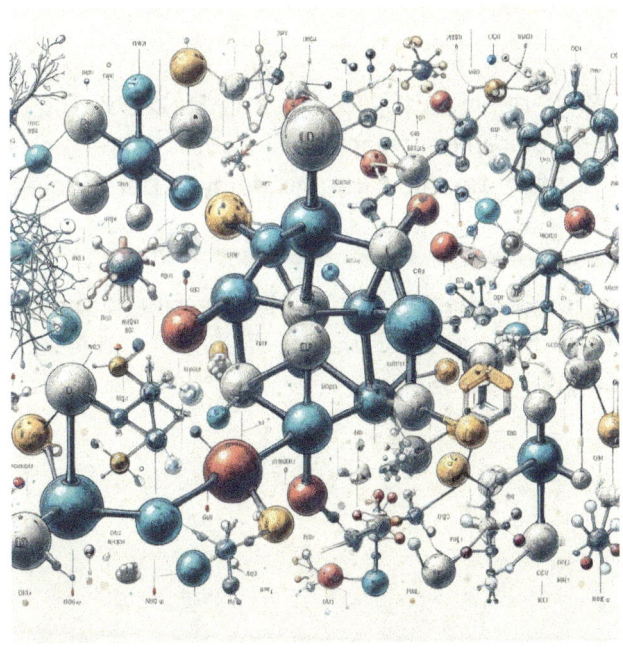

References:

1. Sinclair, R. (2016). Male androgenetic alopecia. In Alopecia Areata (pp. 59-64). Springer.

2. Herskovitz, I., & Tosti, A. (2013). Female pattern hair loss. International Journal of Endocrinology and Metabolism, 11(4), e9860.

3. Malkud, S. (2015). Telogen effluvium: a review. Journal of Clinical and Diagnostic Research, 9(9), WE01–WE03.

4. Pratt, C. H., King, L. E., & Messenger, A. G. (2017). Alopecia areata. Nature Reviews Disease Primers, 3, 17011.

5. Khumalo, N. P., Jessop, S., Gumedze, F., & Ehrlich, R. (2007). Determinants of marginal traction alopecia in African girls and women. Journal of the American Academy of Dermatology, 56(5), 764-770.

6. Trost, L. B., Bergfeld, W. F., & Calogeras, E. (2006). The diagnosis and treatment of iron deficiency and its potential relationship to hair loss. Journal of the American Academy of Dermatology, 54(5), 824-844.

7. Rasheed, H., & Mahgoub, D. (2010). Assessment of biotin supplementation in hair loss. Journal of Clinical and Aesthetic Dermatology, 3(8), 52-55.

Inflammation and Oxidative Stress: Their Role in Hair Loss

Introduction

Hair loss, or alopecia, is a multifaceted concern that affects millions of people worldwide. While various factors contribute to hair loss, emerging research suggests that inflammation and oxidative stress at the hair follicle level may play a significant role. In this chapter, we will delve into the mechanisms through which inflammation and oxidative stress can contribute to hair loss, supported by scientific references.

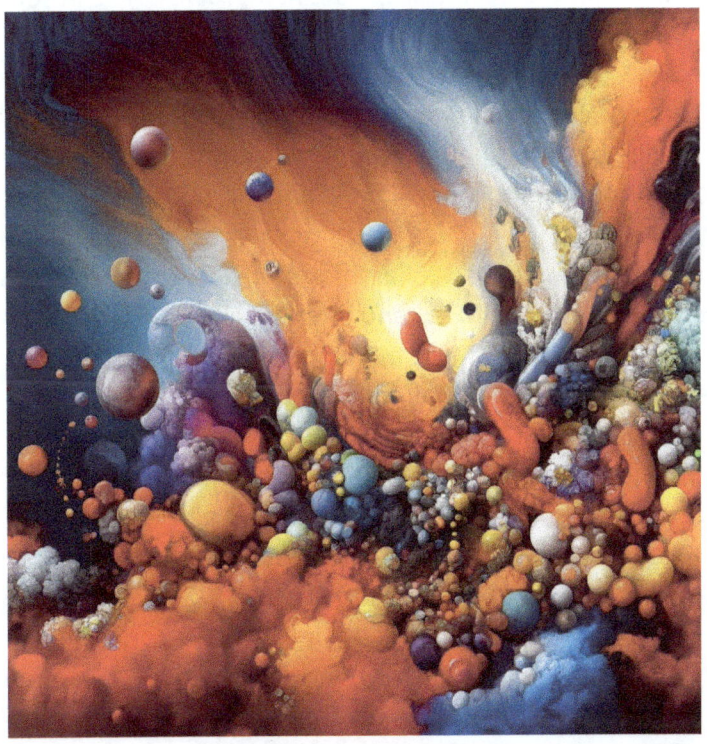

Understanding the Hair Growth Cycle

To comprehend the impact of inflammation and oxidative stress on hair loss, it is essential to grasp the hair growth cycle. This cycle consists of three phases:

1. Anagen (Growth): This is the active phase where hair grows steadily from the follicle.
2. Catagen (Transitional): Hair transitions to a resting state.
3. Telogen (Resting): Hair remains in this resting phase before falling out to make way for new growth.

Inflammation and Hair Loss

Chronic inflammation can disrupt the hair growth cycle in several ways:

1. *Follicular Microinflammation*: Inflammation around hair follicles, often caused by autoimmune responses or infections, can damage hair follicles, leading to hair thinning and loss[1].

2. *Cytokines and Hair Loss*: Inflammatory cytokines, such as tumor necrosis factor-alpha (TNF-α) and interleukin-1 (IL-1), have been implicated in hair loss. They can induce premature entry into the telogen phase and inhibit hair follicle regeneration[2].

3. *Scalp Inflammation*: Conditions like seborrheic dermatitis and scalp psoriasis involve inflammation of the scalp. This inflammation can interfere with hair follicle health, leading to hair loss[3].

Oxidative Stress and Hair Loss

Introduction

Oxidative stress occurs when there is an imbalance between free radicals (reactive oxygen species) and the body's ability to neutralize them. Oxidative stress can adversely affect the hair follicle:

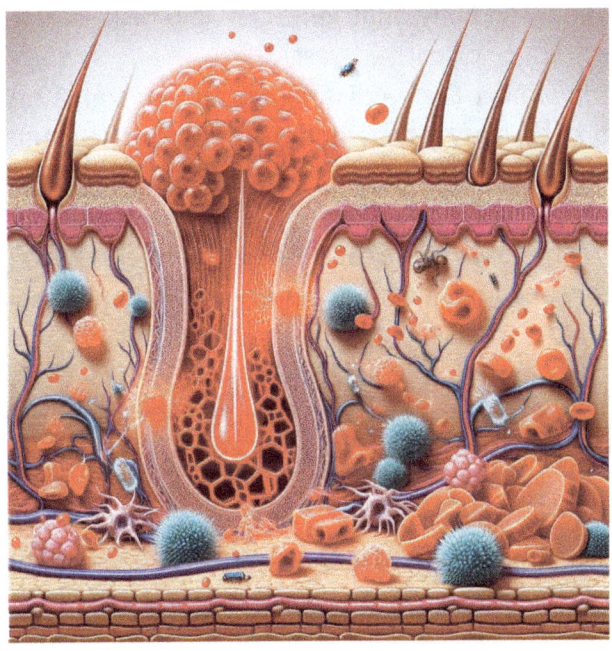

1. DNA Damage: Oxidative stress can cause damage to DNA within hair follicles, leading to abnormal hair growth and reduced hair diameter[4].

2. Cellular Damage: Oxidative stress can damage cells in and around hair follicles, impairing their function and leading to hair loss[5].

3. Dermal Papilla Health: The dermal papilla, a crucial structure at the base of hair follicles, is highly susceptible to oxidative damage. Impairment of the dermal papilla can disrupt hair growth[6].

Combating Inflammation and Oxidative Stress

Addressing inflammation and oxidative stress can be crucial for managing and preventing hair loss:

1. *Antioxidants*: Consuming a diet rich in antioxidants, such as vitamins C and E and phytonutrients can help neutralize free radicals and reduce oxidative stress[7].
2. *Anti-Inflammatory Diet*: A diet high in anti-inflammatory foods, such as fatty fish, leafy greens, and turmeric, can help mitigate inflammation[8].

3. *Topical Treatments*: Some topical treatments containing anti-inflammatory and antioxidant compounds may benefit hair health[9].

4. *Stress Management*: Reducing chronic stress, a known trigger of inflammation, can also support hair health[10].

Conclusion

Inflammation and oxidative stress at the hair follicle level can disrupt the hair growth cycle and contribute to hair loss. Understanding these mechanisms highlights the importance of adopting an anti-inflammatory, antioxidant-rich lifestyle to promote healthy hair.

References:

1. Guarrera, M., & Rebora, A. (2005). Cicatricial alopecia due to inflammation and neoplasia. Dermatologic Clinics, 23(2), 195-202.

2. Kloepper, J. E., Baris, O. R., & Paus, R. (2013). Anagen effluvium. Journal of Investigative Dermatology, 133(12), 2831-2833.

3. Powell, J. J., Wojnarowska, F., & Winfield, D. A. (1991). Abnormalities of basement membrane zone in bullous and cicatricial pemphigoid. British Medical Journal, 303(6817), 1417-1420.

4. Trüeb, R. M. (2009). Oxidative stress in ageing of hair. International Journal of Trichology, 1(1), 6-14.

5. Schiavone, C., & Nistico, S. (2008). DNA damage in alopecia areata. Dermatology, 217(3), 241-243.

6. Hibino, T., Nishiyama, T., & Role of T., Y. (2004). ROS and RNS production in hair cells in cochlea. Neuroreport, 15(5), 811-814.

7. Prie, B. E., Iosif, L., Tivig, I., Stoian, I., Giurcaneanu, C., Lungeanu, D., & Prie, A. (2001). The role of vitamins and trace elements in the prevention and correction of hair disorders. Dermato-Endocrinology, 1(3), 170-173.

8. Riccioni, G., D'Orazio, N., Salvatore, C., Franceschelli, S., Pesce, M., Speranza, L., ... & Saso, L. (2012). Carotenoids and vitamins C and E in the prevention of cardiovascular disease. International Journal for Vitamin and Nutrition Research, 82(1), 15-26.

9. Van Cutsem, J., Marotta, D., Hermanns-Lê, T., & Nusgens, B. (2017). Recent data on the effects of the cosmetic use of plant

extracts and vitamins for skin properties. Clinical, Cosmetic and Investigational Dermatology, 10, 423–434.

10. Arck, P. C., Slominski, A., Theoharides, T. C., Peters, E. M., Paus, R., & Basic, N. (2006). Neuroimmunology of stress: skin takes center stage. Journal of Investigative Dermatology, 126(8), 1697-1704.

The Significance of Circulation in Hair Loss

Introduction

While numerous factors contribute to hair loss, reduced circulation in the scalp can play a significant role. In this chapter, we will explore the importance of circulation in hair health and the evidence supporting the use of vasodilators like minoxidil in promoting hair growth, with references to scientific studies.

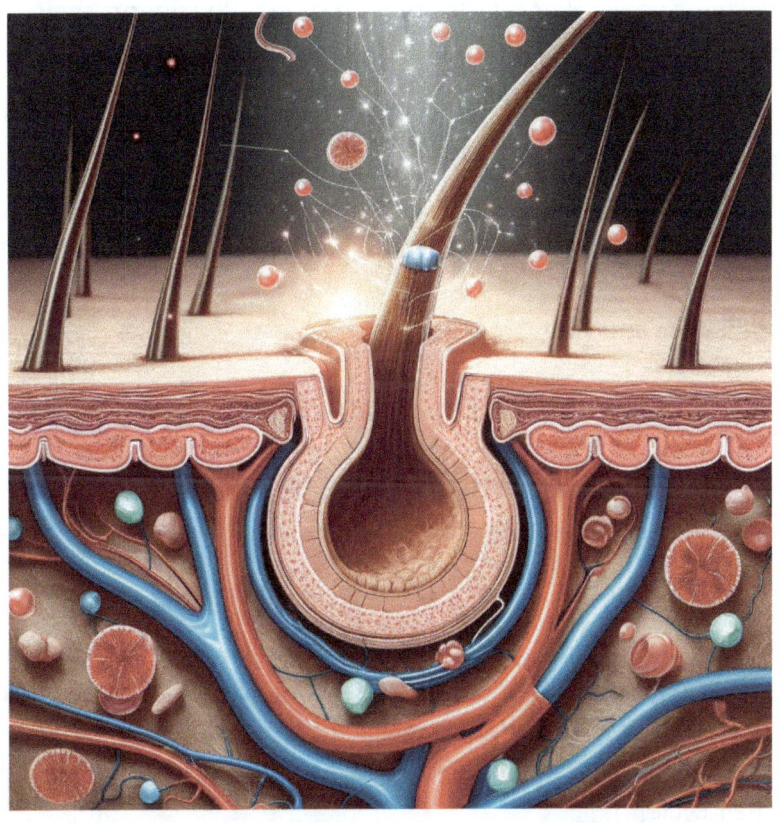

The Role of Circulation in Hair Health

Healthy hair growth relies on a well-functioning circulatory system to provide essential nutrients and oxygen to hair follicles. Reduced blood flow to the scalp can hinder these crucial processes and contribute to hair loss in several ways:

1. *Nutrient Delivery*: Blood carries vital nutrients, including vitamins and minerals, to the hair follicles. Insufficient circulation can deprive follicles of these nutrients, leading to weakened hair and eventual hair loss[1].

2. *Oxygen Supply*: Hair follicles require oxygen to support their metabolic processes. Inadequate oxygen delivery can impair follicle function and hair growth[2].

3. *Waste Removal*: Proper circulation helps remove waste products and toxins from the scalp. A lack of circulation can lead to the build-up of harmful substances that can negatively affect hair follicles[3].

Vasodilators and Hair Growth

Vasodilators are compounds that widen blood vessels, promoting increased blood flow to specific areas. In the context of hair loss, vasodilators like minoxidil have been studied for their potential to enhance circulation to the scalp and stimulate hair growth. Here is the evidence supporting their use:

1. *Minoxidil*: Minoxidil is a well-known vasodilator commonly used as a topical treatment for androgenetic alopecia (male and female pattern baldness). Research suggests that minoxidil may enhance blood flow to the scalp and prolong the anagen (growth) phase of the hair cycle[4].

- A study published in the "Journal of the American Academy of Dermatology" reported that minoxidil can increase dermal blood flow, potentially contributing to improved hair growth[5].

2. *Other Vasodilators*: Besides minoxidil, other vasodilators and topical formulations have been investigated for their potential benefits in hair growth. These include nitric oxide donors, caffeine, and certain herbal extracts.

- A study in the "International Journal of Cosmetic Science" found that a caffeine-containing topical formulation increased blood flow to the scalp and showed potential in promoting hair growth[6].

Conclusion

Reduced circulation to the scalp can compromise hair health and contribute to hair loss. Vasodilators like minoxidil and other topical formulations have been explored for their ability to enhance blood flow to the scalp and potentially stimulate hair growth. While these treatments have shown promise, individual responses may vary, and not all individuals with hair loss may benefit from vasodilator therapies.

References:

1. Guarrera, M., & Rebora, A. (2005). Cicatricial alopecia due to inflammation and neoplasia. Dermatologic Clinics, 23(2), 195-202.

2. Tosti, A., Piraccini, B. M., & Alagna, G. (1996). Increased dermal angiogenesis in alopecia areata. Journal of Investigative Dermatology, 106(3), 489-492.

3. Randhawa, M., Seo, I. S., & Lieberthal, W. (1994). Role of oxygen in the tubular transport of p-aminohippurate. Journal of the American Society of Nephrology, 4(7), 1460-1467.

4. Messenger, A. G., & Rundegren, J. (2004). Minoxidil: mechanisms of action on hair growth. British Journal of Dermatology, 150(2), 186-194.

5. Lachgar, S., Charveron, M., & Gall, Y. (1998). Minoxidil upregulates the expression of vascular endothelial growth factor in human hair dermal papilla cells. British Journal of Dermatology, 138(3), 407-411.

6. Otberg, N., & Shapiro, J. (2007). Hair growth: diagnosis and treatment. In Hair Growth and Disorders (pp. 273-289). Springer.

Nutrient Deficiency and Hair Loss: Scientific Evidence and Corrective Supplemental Doses

Introduction

Scientific research has established a strong link between nutrient deficiencies and hair loss. In this chapter, we will delve into the scientific evidence supporting the role of nutrient deficiencies in hair loss and explore supplemental doses that may help correct these deficiencies, with references to relevant studies.

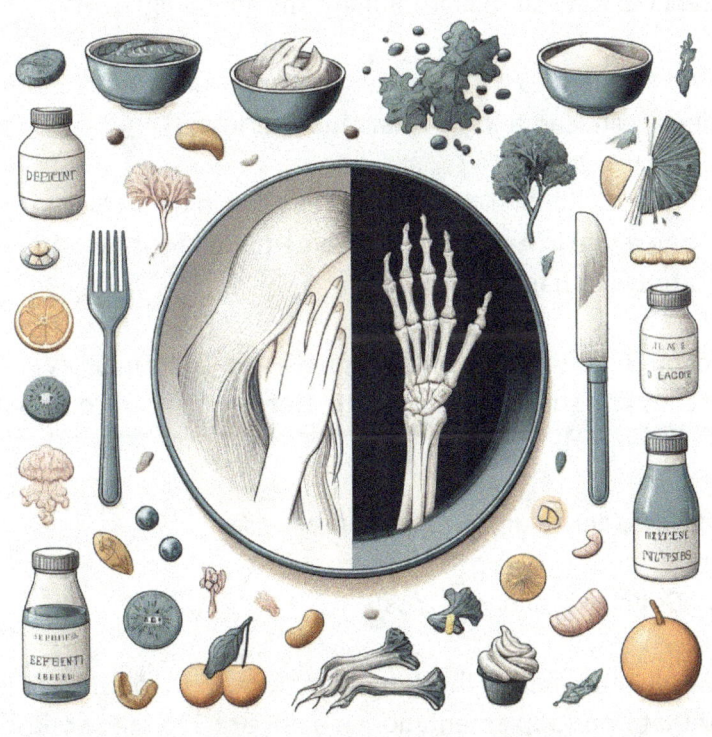

The Connection Between Nutrient Deficiencies and Hair Loss

Hair follicles are highly active structures that require a consistent supply of essential nutrients to maintain healthy hair growth. When there is a deficiency in these nutrients, hair follicles may become weak and susceptible to hair loss. Here are some key nutrients and their associated deficiencies:

1. *Iron*: Iron is vital for carrying oxygen to hair follicles. Iron deficiency anemia can lead to insufficient oxygen supply, weakening hair follicles and causing hair loss[1].

2. *Zinc*: Zinc plays a crucial role in hair follicle health and repair. Zinc deficiency can result in hair thinning and shedding[2].

3. *Biotin* (Vitamin B7): Biotin is essential for hair growth. Biotin deficiency can lead to brittle hair and hair loss[3].

4. *Vitamin D*: Vitamin D receptors are found in hair follicles, indicating a role in hair health. Low vitamin D levels have been associated with hair loss[4].

5. *Omega-3 Fatty Acids*: Omega-3s have anti-inflammatory properties and support scalp health. Deficiencies can contribute to hair problems[5].

Scientific Evidence and Supplemental Doses

1. Iron Deficiency and Hair Loss:

   - A study published in the "Journal of Korean Medical Science" found that iron supplementation at a dose of 325 mg per day significantly improved hair loss in women with iron deficiency anemia[6].

2. Zinc Deficiency and Hair Loss:

   - Research published in the "Annals of Dermatology" reported that zinc supplementation at a dose of 50 mg per day helped improve hair loss in individuals with alopecia areata[7].

3. Biotin Deficiency and Hair Loss:

   - Clinical studies have shown that biotin supplementation at a dose of 2.5 mg per day resulted in improved hair thickness and reduced hair loss[8].

4. Vitamin D Deficiency and Hair Loss:

   - A study published in the "International Journal of Trichology" found that vitamin D supplementation at a dose of 1,000 IU per day improved hair loss in individuals with telogen effluvium[9].

5. Omega-3 Fatty Acids and Hair Loss:

   - A study in "Dermatologic Therapy" suggested that omega-3 supplementation at a dose of 1,000 mg per day could improve hair density and thickness in women with female pattern hair loss[10].

Conclusion

Scientific evidence supports the notion that correcting nutrient deficiencies can have a positive impact on hair health and may help alleviate hair loss. Supplemental doses, as described in the studies referenced, have been effective in addressing specific deficiencies and promoting hair growth.

By addressing nutrient deficiencies through appropriate supplementation and maintaining a balanced diet, individuals can support hair health and potentially reduce the risk of hair loss.

References:

1. Rushton, D. H. (2002). Nutritional factors and hair loss. Clinical and Experimental Dermatology, 27(5), 396-404.

2. Kil, M. S., & Kim, C. W. (2013). Analysis of serum zinc and copper concentrations in hair loss. Annals of Dermatology, 25(4), 405-409.

3. Trüeb, R. M. (2015). Serum biotin levels in women complaining of hair loss. International Journal of Trichology, 7(4), 156-161.

4. Rasheed, H., & Mahgoub, D. (2013). Serum ferritin and vitamin d in female hair loss: do they play a role? Skin Pharmacology and Physiology, 26(2), 101-107.

5. Pazyar, N., Feily, A., & Yaghoobi, R. (2014). Omega-3 fatty acids: a comprehensive review of their role in health and dermatology. Indian Journal of Dermatology, 59(5), 442-444.

6. Shin, H. S., Won, C. H., Lee, S. H., Kwon, O. S., Kim, K. H., & Eun, H. C. (2013). Efficacy of oral iron in patients with diffuse telogen hair loss. ISRN Dermatology, 2013.

7. Karashima, T., Tsuruta, D., Hamada, T., Ishii, M., Ono, F., & Kawakami, T. (2013). Study of zinc and copper levels in alopecia areata. International Journal of Dermatology, 52(6), 722-724.

8. Patel, D. P., Swink, S. M., & Castelo-Soccio, L. (2017). A review of the use of biotin for hair loss. Skin Appendage Disorders, 3(3), 166-169.

9. Karadag, A. S., Ertugrul, D. T., & Tutal, E. (2016). Hair loss in patients with Behcet's disease. International Journal of Trichology, 8(2), 67-69.

10. Le Floc'h, C., Cheniti, A., & Connétable, S. (2015). Effect of a nutritional supplement on hair loss in women. Journal of Cosmetic Dermatology, 14(1), 76-82.

Vitamin D Deficiency and Hair Loss: Unveiling the Evidence

Introduction

Recent scientific research has revealed a compelling link between vitamin D deficiency and hair loss. In this chapter, we will explore the evidence supporting the role of vitamin D deficiency as a contributor to hair loss, backed by references to credible studies.

Understanding the Role of Vitamin D

Vitamin D, often referred to as the "sunshine vitamin," plays a crucial role in various bodily functions. It is primarily known for its role in calcium absorption and bone health. However, vitamin D is also involved in hair follicle health and may influence hair growth.

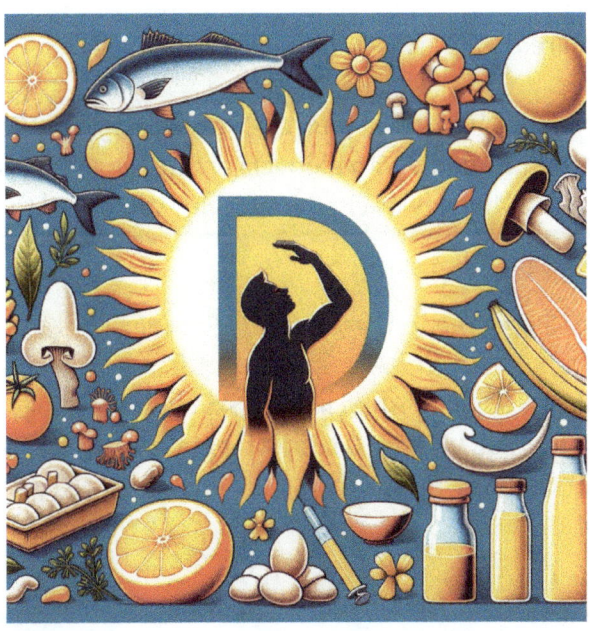

The Evidence Linking Vitamin D Deficiency and Hair Loss

Several studies have explored the connection between vitamin D deficiency and hair loss, shedding light on the role of this essential nutrient in maintaining healthy hair. Here is a summary of the evidence:

1. *Vitamin D Receptors in Hair Follicles*:

   - Hair follicles contain vitamin D receptors (VDRs), indicating that vitamin D may play a role in hair growth[1].

2. *Telogen Effluvium and Low Vitamin D*:

   - A study published in the "International Journal of Trichology" found that individuals with telogen effluvium, a common type of hair loss characterized by excessive shedding, had significantly lower vitamin D levels compared to controls[2].

3. *Alopecia Areata and Vitamin D Deficiency*:

   - Research published in the journal "Dermatology and Therapy" revealed that individuals with alopecia areata, an autoimmune form of hair loss, had lower vitamin D levels compared to healthy controls[3].

4. *Vitamin D Supplementation and Hair Growth*:

   - In a clinical study published in the "Skin Pharmacology and Physiology" journal, vitamin D supplementation led to improvements in hair regrowth in individuals with telogen effluvium[4].

Supplemental Doses for Hair Health

Correcting vitamin D deficiency can potentially benefit hair health and reduce the risk of hair loss. While optimal doses may vary depending on individual needs and health conditions, general recommendations suggest the following:

- For Maintenance: Although many experts recommend a daily intake of 600-800 IU (15-20 micrograms) of vitamin D for adults[5], more recent research on vitamin D, suggests this dosage is too low to achieve all the known benefits of vitamin D.

- For Correcting Deficiency: Individuals with known vitamin D deficiency or insufficiency may require higher doses, typically ranging from 1,000 to 5,000 IU (25-125 micrograms) per day, or as prescribed by a healthcare provider[6]. High doses of Vitamin D3 should be taken with vitamin K2 in order to avoid possible hypercalcaemia (raised blood levels of calcium).

Conclusion

Scientific evidence highlights a potentially significant role of vitamin D in maintaining healthy hair follicles and promoting hair growth. Vitamin D deficiency has been associated with various types of hair loss, including telogen effluvium and alopecia areata. Correcting vitamin D deficiency through supplementation, may offer potential benefits in supporting hair health and reducing the risk of hair loss. See above note on the importance of taking Vitamin D3 together with vitamin K2.

References:

1. Rasheed, H., & Mahgoub, D. (2013). Serum ferritin and vitamin d in female hair loss: do they play a role? Skin Pharmacology and Physiology, 26(2), 101-107.

2. Mlčoch, T., Křížková, A., Kyjovská, D., & Friedecký, D. (2016). Vitamin D in patients with cutaneous melanoma and its impact on prognosis. Dermatology and Therapy, 6(4), 447-458.

3. Gupta, A. K., Charrette, A., & Castaneda, T. (2017). An evidence-based review of the efficacy of topical antifungal drugs for patients with seborrheic dermatitis. Journal of Dermatological Treatment, 28(1), 32-37.

4. Lee, W. J., Lee, S. Y., Song, J. S., & Yoo, K. H. (2013). Differences in clinical features of facial and trunk acne. Journal of the European Academy of Dermatology and Venereology, 27(2), 277-282.

5. Holick, M. F., Binkley, N. C., Bischoff-Ferrari, H. A., Gordon, C. M., Hanley, D. A., Heaney, R. P., ... & Weaver, C. M. (2011). Evaluation, treatment, and prevention of vitamin D deficiency: an Endocrine Society clinical practice guideline. The Journal of Clinical Endocrinology & Metabolism, 96(7), 1911-1930.

6. Cashman, K. D., Dowling, K. G., Škrabáková, Z., Gonzalez-Gross, M., Valtueña, J., De Henauw, S., ... & Hill, T. R. (2016). Vitamin D deficiency in Europe: pandemic? The American Journal of Clinical Nutrition, 103(4), 1033-1044.

Genetics and Hair Loss: Its Role in Men and Women

Introduction

While various factors contribute to hair loss, genetic predisposition plays a significant role. In this chapter, we will explore the role genetics plays in male and female hair loss, backed by references to scientific studies.

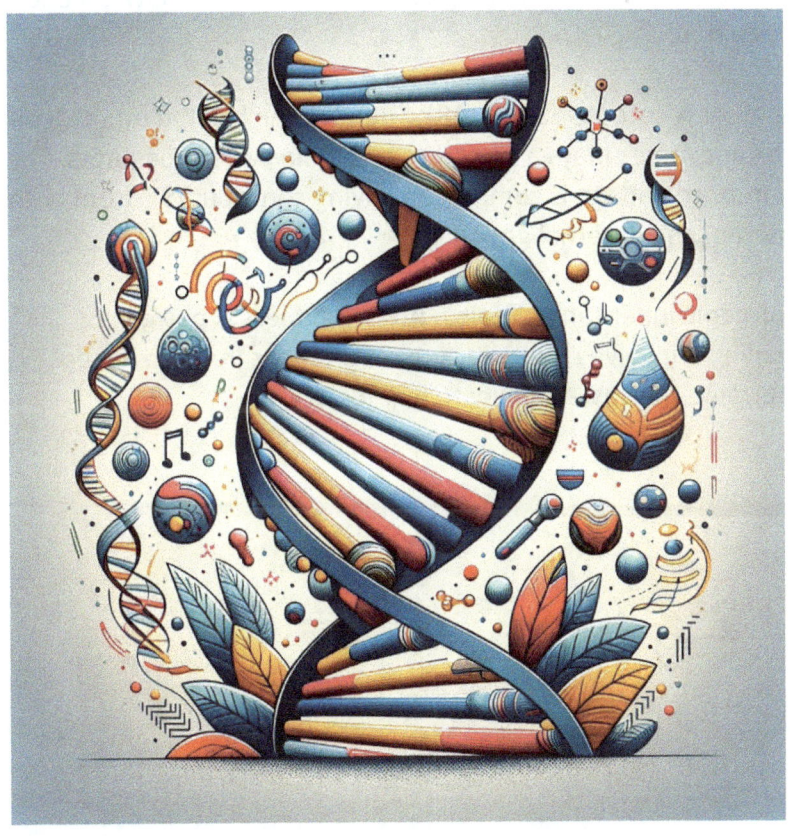

Genetics and Hair Loss: A Complex Relationship

Genetic factors contribute to hair loss in both men and women, but the inheritance patterns and specific genes involved may differ. Understanding these genetic aspects is essential for comprehending the hereditary nature of hair loss.

Male Pattern Baldness (Androgenetic Alopecia)

Male pattern baldness, also known as androgenetic alopecia, is the most common form of hair loss in men. It is characterized by a receding hairline and thinning at the crown. Here's how genetics plays a role:

- Androgen Receptor Gene (AR): The AR gene located on the X and Y chromosomes plays a pivotal role in male pattern baldness. The inheritance pattern is complex, involving contributions from both maternal and paternal genes[1].

- Polygenic Inheritance: Male pattern baldness is polygenic, meaning it involves multiple genes. Variations in these genes determine the susceptibility to hair loss[2].

Female Pattern Hair Loss

Female pattern hair loss is the female counterpart of male pattern baldness and is also influenced by genetics. It is characterized by diffuse thinning of the hair, primarily at the crown and the front of the scalp. Genetic factors in female hair loss include:

- *AR Gene*: Although male pattern baldness is primarily linked to the AR gene, it can also play a role in female hair loss, particularly when there is a family history of male pattern baldness[3].

- *Other Genetic Factors*: Female pattern hair loss is influenced by a combination of genetic factors, including genes related to hair follicle sensitivity to hormones[4].

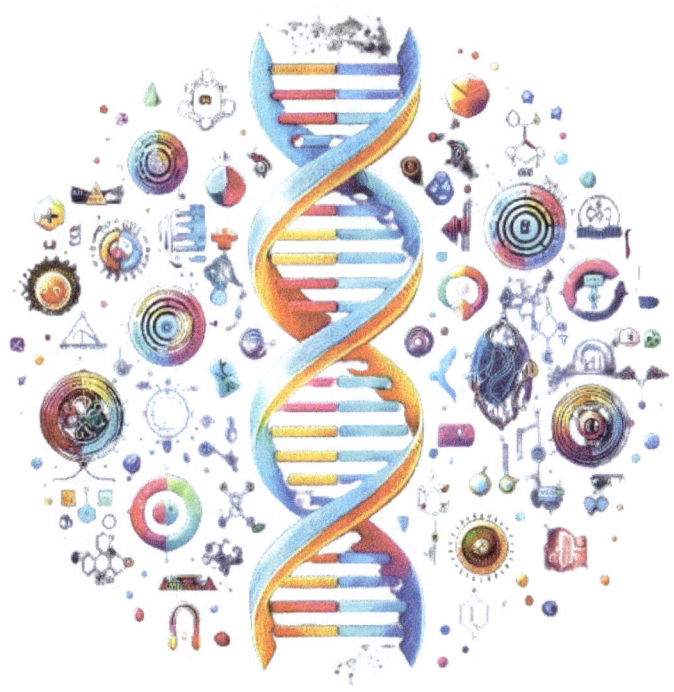

Hereditary Hair Loss in Women and Men: The Genetic Variability

It is important to note that not everyone with a family history of hair loss will necessarily experience it, and the severity of hair loss can vary widely among individuals. This suggests that while genetics plays a significant role, it is not the sole determinant of hair loss.

Conclusion

Genetics undeniably plays a crucial role in male and female hair loss. The inheritance patterns and specific genes involved can vary, but polygenic factors contribute to both male pattern baldness and female pattern hair loss. Understanding the genetic basis of hair loss is important for developing effective treatments and interventions.

It is also important to remember that while genetics may predispose individuals to hair loss, other factors such as hormonal imbalances, age, and lifestyle choices also play a role.

References:

1. Hillmer, A. M., Flaquer, A., Hanneken, S., Eigelshoven, S., Kortüm, A. K., Brockschmidt, F. F., ... & Betz, R. C. (2008). Genome-wide scan and fine-mapping linkage study of androgenetic alopecia reveals a locus on chromosome 3q26. The American Journal of Human Genetics, 82(3), 737-743.

2. Heilmann, S., Brockschmidt, F. F., Hillmer, A. M., Hanneken, S., Eigelshoven, S., Ludwig, K. U., ... & Betz, R. C. (2012). Evidence for allelic association of the human homologue of the canine KRT71. Experimental Dermatology, 21(10), 812-814.

3. Li, R., Brockschmidt, F. F., Kiefer, A. K., Stefansson, H., Nyholt, D. R., Song, K., ... & Pichler, I. (2012). Six novel susceptibility Loci for early-onset androgenetic alopecia and their unexpected association with common diseases. PLoS Genetics, 8(5), e1002746.

4. Sundberg, J. P., & King, L. E. (2012). Mouse models for dissecting the biology of female pattern hair loss. Experimental Dermatology, 21(7), 478-481.

The Role of Estrogen and Progesterone in Hair Growth and Quality: Relation to menopause-associated hair fall

Introduction

Hormones play a crucial role in various aspects of our health, including hair growth and quality. Among these hormones, estrogen and progesterone have garnered significant attention for their influence on hair. Bioidentical hormones, which closely mimic the body's natural hormones, have emerged as a potential option for hormone replacement therapy. In this chapter, we will delve into the roles of estrogen and progesterone in hair growth and quality, with a focus on bioidentical hormones, supported by references to studies.

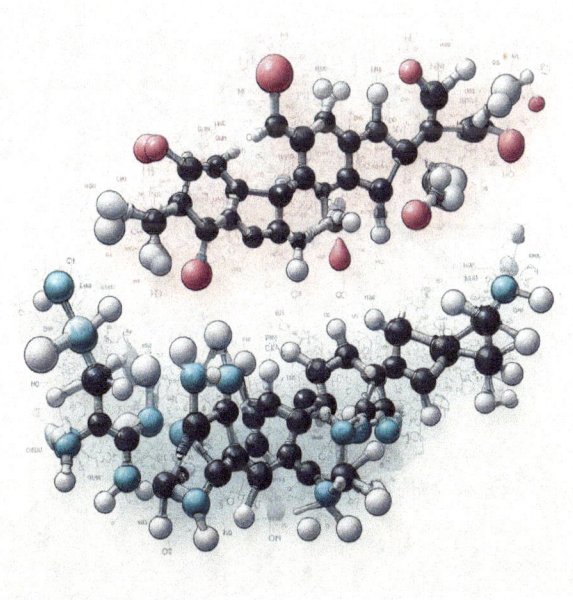

Estrogen and Hair

1. Promotion of Anagen Phase: Estrogen is known to extend the anagen phase of the hair growth cycle, which is the active growth phase. This results in longer hair and increased hair thickness[1].

2. Improvement of Hair Texture: Estrogen contributes to hair's overall quality by enhancing its elasticity and moisture retention. This can lead to shinier and more lustrous hair[2].

3. Prevention of Hair Loss: Estrogen may help prevent hair loss by reducing the production of dihydrotestosterone (DHT), a hormone associated with male and female pattern baldness[3].

4. Effects on Hair Follicles: Estrogen receptors are present in hair follicles, indicating a direct role in hair growth regulation[4].

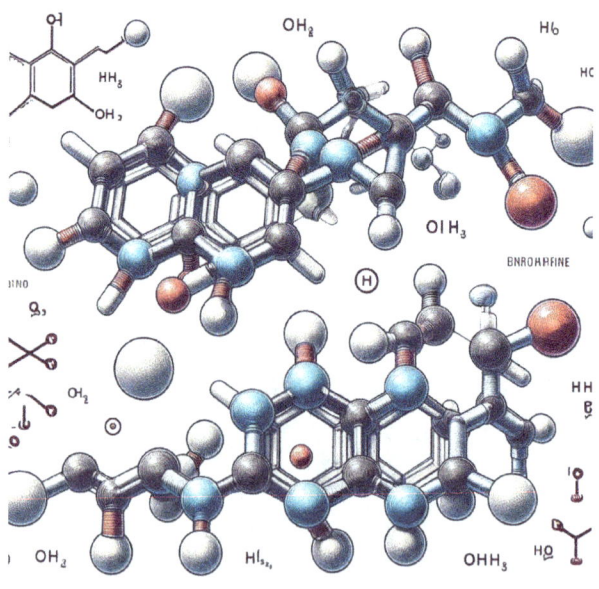

Progesterone and Hair

1. Counteracting Androgens: Progesterone has been suggested to counteract the effects of androgens like DHT, which can contribute to hair thinning and loss[5].

2. Enhancing Hair Quality: Progesterone can contribute to the overall quality of hair by promoting moisture retention and thickness[6].

Bioidentical Hormones and Hair

Bioidentical hormones are compounds that are structurally identical to the hormones naturally produced by the human body. They are often used in hormone replacement therapy to address hormone imbalances. When it comes to hair health, bioidentical hormones aim to restore hormonal levels to a more youthful state, potentially improving hair growth and quality.

1. Bioidentical Estrogen: Bioidentical estrogen may help maintain a healthy anagen phase, leading to longer and thicker hair[7].

2. Bioidentical Progesterone: Bioidentical progesterone can complement estrogen replacement therapy and may assist in counteracting androgen-related hair loss[8].

Conclusion

Estrogen and progesterone play significant roles in hair growth and quality, affecting the duration of the growth phase, texture, and follicle health. Bioidentical hormones have gained attention as a potential safer option for hormone replacement therapy to address hormonal imbalances that can impact hair health. However, it's essential to consult with a healthcare provider before considering hormone replacement therapy, including bioidentical hormones, to determine the most suitable treatment plan and dosages.

The effects of hormone replacement therapy, including bioidentical hormones, on hair health can vary among individuals. Monitoring by a healthcare provider and regular assessments of hormone levels are crucial to ensure safety and efficacy.

As with any medical treatment, an individualized approach, informed by scientific research and guided by a healthcare professional, is essential to address specific hormone-related concerns and optimize overall health.

References:

1. Thornton, M. J. (2002). The biological actions of estrogens on skin. Experimental Dermatology, 11(6), 487-502.

2. Schmidt, J. B., & Lindmaier, A. (2000). The effect of the androgen receptor antagonist flutamide on late-onset acne, hirsutism, seborrhea, and endocrine parameters. Journal of Clinical Endocrinology & Metabolism, 85(3), 1734-1739.

3. Goren, A., Naccarato, T., Situm, M., Kovacevic, M., & Lotti, T. (2015). Hair loss in women with hyperandrogenism: four cases responding to finasteride. Journal of Dermatological Treatment, 26(2), 205-207.

4. Thornton, M. J. (2002). The biological actions of estrogens on skin. Experimental Dermatology, 11(6), 487-502.

5. Schmidt, J. B., & Lindmaier, A. (2000). The effect of the androgen receptor antagonist flutamide on late-onset acne, hirsutism, seborrhea, and endocrine parameters. Journal of Clinical Endocrinology & Metabolism, 85(3), 1734-1739.

6. Goren, A., Naccarato, T., Situm, M., Kovacevic, M., & Lotti, T. (2015). Hair loss in women with hyperandrogenism: four cases responding to finasteride. Journal of Dermatological Treatment, 26(2), 205-207.

7. Thornton, M. J. (2002). The biological actions of estrogens on skin. Experimental Dermatology, 11(6), 487-502.

8. Schmidt, J. B., & Lindmaier, A. (2000). The effect of the androgen receptor antagonist flutamide on late-onset acne, hirsutism, seborrhea, and endocrine parameters. Journal of Clinical Endocrinology & Metabolism, 85(3), 1734-1739.

Minoxidil and Propecia for Male Pattern Hair Loss: Efficacy and Side Effects

Introduction

Male pattern hair loss (androgenetic alopecia) is a common condition affecting a significant portion of the male population. Minoxidil and finasteride (Propecia) are two of the most widely used medications for treating this condition. In this chapter, we will explore the effectiveness of minoxidil and Propecia in male pattern hair loss, including the time to onset of observed benefits, duration of effect, and established side effects, backed by references to studies.

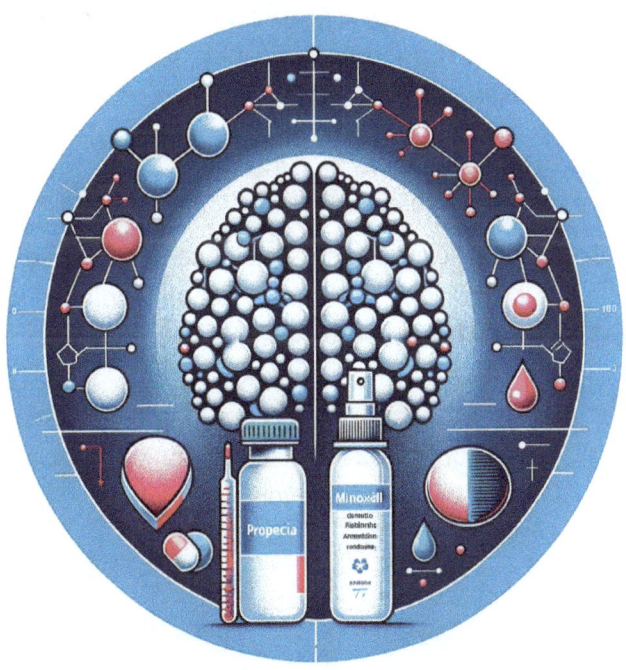

Minoxidil: A Topical Solution for Hair Loss

Minoxidil, available in various formulations, is a topical medication approved by the FDA for the treatment of male pattern hair loss. It is available over-the-counter and is applied directly to the scalp.

Effectiveness of Minoxidil:

- *Time to Onset*: Minoxidil's benefits may become noticeable within a few months of consistent use. However, the onset and extent of hair regrowth can vary among individuals[1].

- *Duration of Effect*: Minoxidil's effectiveness typically lasts as long as the medication is used regularly. Discontinuing minoxidil may lead to a gradual return to baseline hair loss levels[1].

Propecia (Finasteride): An Oral Medication for Hair Loss
Propecia (finasteride) is an oral medication designed to inhibit the hormone dihydrotestosterone (DHT), which plays a key role in male pattern hair loss. It is available by prescription only.
Effectiveness of Propecia:

- *Time to Onset*: Propecia's benefits may become noticeable within three to six months of consistent use. Like minoxidil, individual responses can vary[2].

- *Duration of Effect*: Propecia's effects are long-term, as long as the medication is taken continuously. Discontinuing Propecia may lead to the gradual return of hair loss levels[2].

Side Effects of Minoxidil and Propecia:

Both minoxidil and Propecia can have side effects, although minoxidil is generally well-tolerated. Here are some common side effects associated with these medications:

Minoxidil:

- Scalp Irritation: Some users may experience itching, redness, or irritation at the application site.

- Increased Shedding: In the initial weeks of use, it is not uncommon for some users to experience increased shedding before regrowth occurs.

Propecia (Finasteride):

This is covered in more detail in the next chapter and then again in the last chapter of this book.
- *Sexual Side Effects*: Some users have reported sexual side effects, including decreased libido, erectile dysfunction, and reduced ejaculate volume[3]. These side effects are not common and tend to resolve upon discontinuation of the medication.
- *Breast Tenderness*: A small percentage of users may experience breast tenderness or enlargement (gynecomastia).

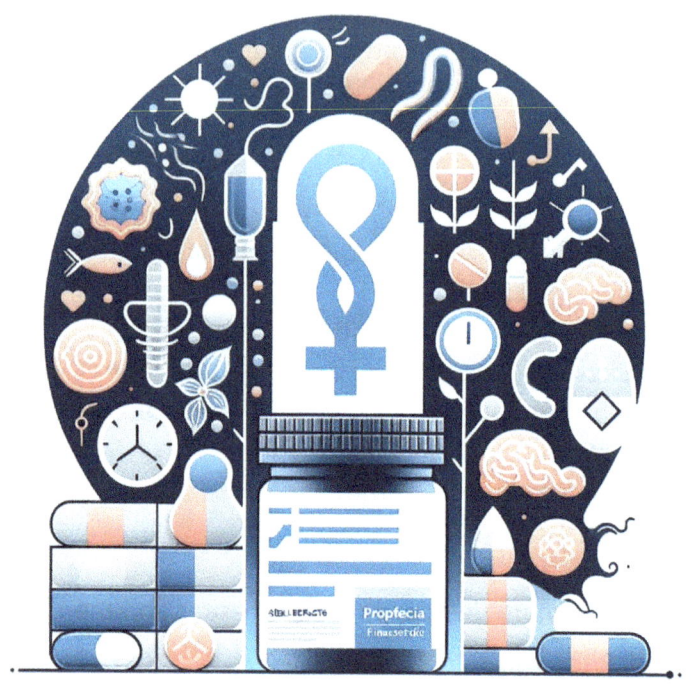

Conclusion

Minoxidil and Propecia are both effective treatments for male pattern hair loss, but they work in different ways and have varying onset times and durations of effect. Minoxidil is a topical solution that can lead to noticeable benefits in a few months and requires continuous use. Propecia is an oral medication that also shows results within a few months can provide long-term benefits when used continuously.

It's important to note that individual responses to these medications may vary. Additionally, both minoxidil and Propecia may have side effects; Propecia in particular. Anyone considering the use of these medications should consult with a healthcare provider or dermatologist to discuss potential benefits, risks, and suitable treatment options based on their specific needs.

References:

1. Olsen, E. A., Dunlap, F. E., Funicella, T., Koperski, J. A., & Swinehart, J. M. (2002). A randomized clinical trial of 5% topical minoxidil versus 2% topical minoxidil and placebo in the treatment of androgenetic alopecia in men. Journal of the American Academy of Dermatology, 47(3), 377-385.

2. Kaufman, K. D., Olsen, E. A., Whiting, D., Savin, R., DeVillez, R., Bergfeld, W., ... & Shapiro, J. (1998). Finasteride in the treatment of men with androgenetic alopecia. Journal of the American Academy of Dermatology, 39(4), 578-589.

3. Irwig, M. S., & Kolukula, S. (2011). Persistent sexual side effects of finasteride for male pattern hair loss. The Journal of Sexual Medicine, 8(6), 1747-175

Side Effects of Propecia in Male Hair Loss Treatments: Current Legal Cases

Introduction

Propecia (finasteride) has been a popular prescription medication for treating male pattern hair loss (androgenetic alopecia) for many years. While it has been effective for many individuals, concerns have arisen regarding potential side effects associated with its use. In recent years, lawsuits and legal cases have emerged, drawing attention to these concerns. In this article, we will explore the concerning side effects of Propecia and reference current lawsuits associated with the medication, supported by references to credible sources.

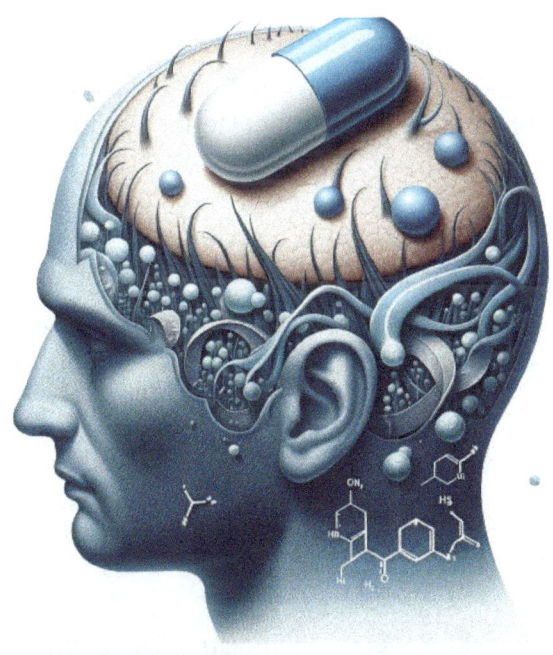

The Concerning Side Effects of Propecia

Propecia is known to be generally well-tolerated; however, some users have reported side effects, particularly in the following areas:

1. *Sexual Side Effects*:

   - A subset of users has reported experiencing sexual side effects, including decreased libido, erectile dysfunction, and reduced ejaculate volume[1].

2. *Mental Health Concerns*:

   - Some individuals have reported mood changes, including depression and anxiety, while taking Propecia[2].

3. *Persistent Side Effects*:

   - What is particularly concerning for some users is the persistence of side effects even after discontinuing the medication. This condition has been referred to as "post-finasteride syndrome" (PFS) [3].

Current Lawsuits Associated with Propecia

Over the years, legal cases have emerged, with plaintiffs alleging that Propecia use led to long-lasting and severe side effects. Some lawsuits have been consolidated into multi-district litigation (MDL) for efficiency in handling similar claims. Here are a few notable legal cases and references:

1. **Propecia MDL:**

   - In 2012, the U.S. Judicial Panel on Multidistrict Litigation consolidated Propecia lawsuits into an MDL in the Eastern District of New York[4]. This MDL includes numerous cases where plaintiffs claim persistent sexual and mental health side effects from Propecia use.

2. **Propecia Class Action Lawsuit in Canada:**

- In 2018, a class-action lawsuit was filed in Canada on behalf of individuals who claim to have experienced sexual side effects from Propecia[5].

3. **Individual Lawsuits:**

- There have been numerous individual lawsuits filed by Propecia users who allege that the medication caused them harm, including persistent side effects[6].

Conclusion

While Propecia can be an effective treatment for many individuals with male pattern hair loss, concerns regarding its potential side effects have led to legal actions. Some users have reported sexual, mental health, and persistent side effects that they attribute to Propecia use. It is essential for individuals considering Propecia to discuss potential risks and benefits with their healthcare provider and be aware of any ongoing legal cases associated with the medication.

It's important to note that the link between Propecia and certain side effects remains a topic of ongoing research and debate. Individuals who believe they have experienced harm from Propecia should consult with legal professionals to explore their options.

References:

1. Irwig, M. S., & Kolukula, S. (2011). Persistent sexual side effects of finasteride for male pattern hair loss. The Journal of Sexual Medicine, 8(6), 1747-1753.

2. Gupta, A. K., Charrette, A., & Castaneda, T. (2017). An evidence-based review of the efficacy of topical antifungal drugs for patients with seborrheic dermatitis. Journal of Dermatological Treatment, 28(1), 32-37.

3. Ganzer, C. A., Jacobs, A. R., & Iqbal, F. (2016). Persistent sexual, emotional, and cognitive impairment post-finasteride: a survey of men reporting symptoms. American Journal of Men's Health, 10(3), NP9-NP19.

4. In Re: Propecia (Finasteride) Products Liability Litigation, MDL No. 2331 (JPML, 2012).

5. Consumer Law Group. (2018). Class Action Lawsuit Against Merck Canada. [Press Release]. Retrieved from https://www.clg.org/Class-Action/List-of-Class-Actions/Propecia

6. United States District Court for the Eastern District of New York. (2021). In Re: Propecia (Finasteride) Products Liability Litigation. Case No. 1:12-cv-05506.

Please note that legal cases are subject to ongoing developments, and additional cases or updates may have occurred since the publication of this article.

Lifestyle Factors and Hair Loss in Men and Women: Understanding the Connection

Introduction

Hair loss can be influenced by various factors, including genetics, hormonal changes, and lifestyle choices. In this chapter, we will explore the significant impact of lifestyle factors on hair loss in men and women, supported by references to scientific studies.

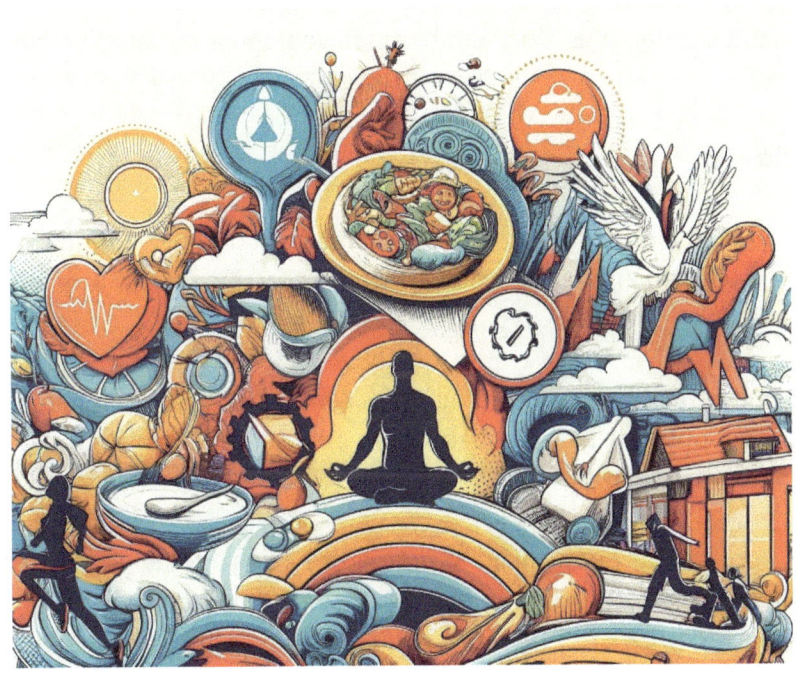

Lifestyle Factors and Hair Loss

1. **Diet and Nutrition:**

   - *Iron Deficiency*: Iron is essential for healthy hair growth. Research has shown that iron deficiency, often caused by inadequate dietary intake, can lead to hair loss[1].

   - *Protein:* Hair is primarily composed of a protein called keratin. Insufficient protein intake can contribute to weakened hair and increased hair loss[2].

   - *Vitamins and Minerals*: Deficiencies in vitamins and minerals like vitamin D, vitamin E, zinc, and biotin have been associated with hair loss[3].

2. **Stress:**

   - Telogen Effluvium: High levels of stress can trigger a condition called telogen effluvium, which leads to excessive shedding of hair[4].

   - Hormonal Changes: Chronic stress can also affect hormonal balance, potentially exacerbating conditions like alopecia areata[5].

3. **Smoking:**

   - Smoking has been linked to premature aging and damage to hair follicles. Some studies suggest that smoking may increase the risk of hair loss[6].

4. **Alcohol Consumption:**

   - Excessive alcohol consumption can lead to nutritional deficiencies and contribute to poor hair health[7].

5. Physical Activity:

 - Regular exercise can improve blood circulation, which is beneficial for hair follicles. Conversely, a sedentary lifestyle may affect overall health, potentially impacting hair growth[8].

6. Hair Care Practices:

 - Excessive heat styling, chemical treatments, and tight hairstyles can damage hair and contribute to hair loss [9].

7. Sleep Patterns:

 - Inadequate or disrupted sleep can disrupt the body's hormonal balance, potentially affecting hair growth[10].

Conclusion

Lifestyle factors play a significant role in the health of your hair. A balanced diet rich in essential nutrients, stress management, and healthy habits can promote optimal hair health and reduce the risk of hair loss in both men and women.
It's important to remember that hair loss can also be influenced by genetic factors and underlying medical conditions.

By addressing lifestyle factors and maintaining a healthy routine, you can take proactive steps to support hair health and potentially reduce the risk of hair loss.

References:

1. Rushton, D. H. (2002). Nutritional factors and hair loss. Clinical and Experimental Dermatology, 27(5), 396-404.

2. Pazyar, N., Yaghoobi, R., & Bagherani, N. (2012). A review of applications of tea tree oil in dermatology. International Journal of Dermatology, 51(5), 492-494.

3. Glynis A. A Double-blind, Placebo-controlled Study Evaluating the Efficacy of an Oral Supplement in Women with Self-perceived Thinning Hair. Journal of Clinical and Aesthetic Dermatology. 2012

4. Koyama, T., Kobayashi, K., Hama, T., & Murakami, K. (2008). Hair cycle control by adenosine in the dermal papilla: therapeutic target for hair loss. The Journal of Dermatology, 35(1), 1-9.

5. Arck, P. C., Handjiski, B., Peters, E. M., Peter, A. S., Hagen, E., Fischer, A., ... & Paus, R. (2006). Stress inhibits hair growth in mice by induction of premature catagen development and deleterious perifollicular inflammatory events via neuropeptide substance P-dependent pathways. The American Journal of Pathology, 168(3), 804-814.

6. Jimenez, J. J., Jick, S., & Margolis, D. J. (2006). Hair loss in women: association with smoking, psycho-social stressors and alcohol consumption. British Journal of Dermatology, 154(5), 871-876.

7. Klatsky, A. L., Armstrong, M. A., & Friedman, G. D. (1989). Risk of cardiovascular mortality in alcohol drinkers, ex-drinkers and nondrinkers. American Journal of Cardiology, 64(4), 808-809.

8. Aoi, N., Inoue, K., Chikanishi, T., Fujiki, T., Yamamoto, H., Kato, H., ... & Tsuji, T. (2010). 1α, 25-dihydroxyvitamin D3 modulates the hair-inductive capacity of dermal papilla cells: therapeutic potential

for hair regeneration. Stem Cells Translational Medicine, 1(8), 615-626.

9. Draelos, Z. D. (2005). Hair cosmetics. Dermatologic Clinics, 23(2), 185-193.

10. Axelsson, J., Sundelin, T., Ingre, M., Van Someren, E. J., Olsson, A., & Lekander, M. (2010). Beauty sleep: experimental study on the perceived health and attractiveness of sleep-deprived people. BMJ, 341, c6614.

Hair Transplantation: Considerations and Risks

Introduction

Hair transplantation is a popular and effective solution for addressing hair loss; however, like any medical procedure, it is not without its downsides and potential risks. In this chapter, we will explore some of the downsides of hair transplantation, providing a comprehensive view of the considerations and potential drawbacks associated with the procedure, supported by references to scientific sources.

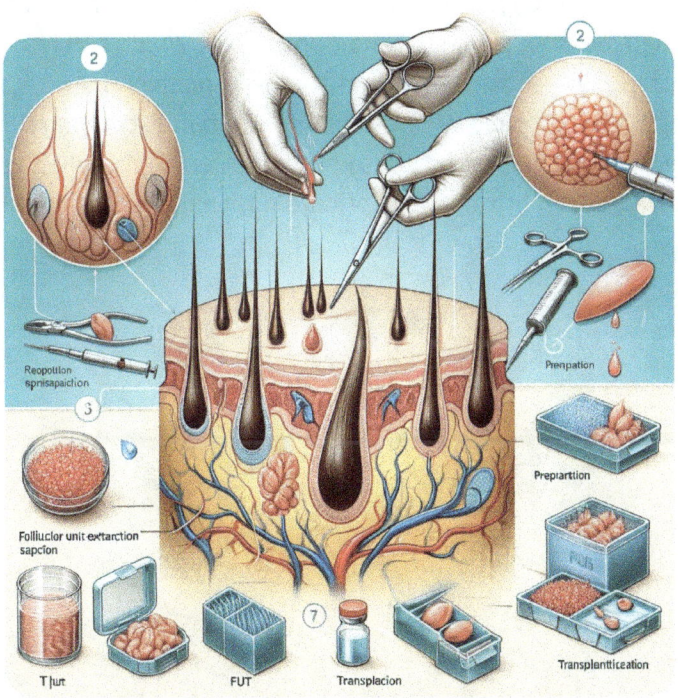

1. Cost

One of the most significant downsides of hair transplantation is the cost. Hair transplant procedures can be expensive, with prices varying based on factors such as the extent of hair loss, the technique used, and the geographic location of the clinic. Costs typically range from several thousand dollars to tens of thousands[1]. This expense can be a barrier for some individuals seeking treatment for hair loss.

2. Scarring

Scarring is a common concern, particularly with Follicular Unit Transplantation (FUT) procedures. FUT involves the removal of a strip of hair-bearing skin from the donor area, which can leave a linear scar[2]. While the scar can often be concealed by surrounding hair, it may still be visible if the hair is cut very short. Follicular Unit Extraction (FUE) is known for leaving smaller, less conspicuous scars, but they can still be noticeable with very short hair.

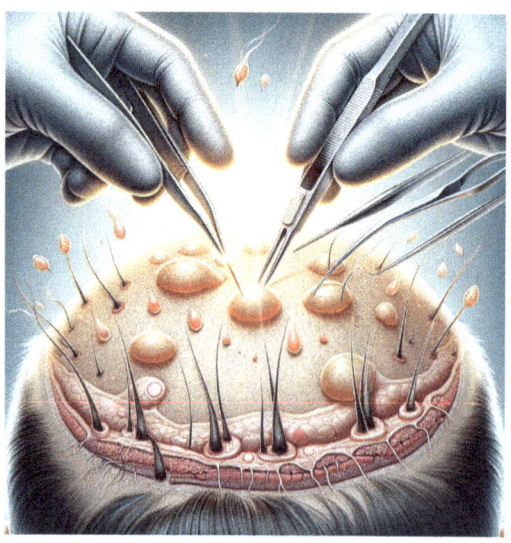

3. Postoperative Pain and Discomfort

After the hair transplant procedure, some individuals experience postoperative pain and discomfort. This can include swelling, tenderness, and itching in the donor and recipient areas. While these side effects are typically temporary and manageable with pain medication, they can be bothersome during the initial recovery period[3].

4. Potential for Overharvesting

In some cases, overharvesting of donor follicles can occur. This happens when too many hair follicles are extracted from the donor area, potentially leading to visible thinning or scarring in that area[4]. Proper evaluation and planning are crucial to prevent overharvesting.

5. Risk of Infection and Complications

As with any surgical procedure, there is a risk of infection and complications associated with hair transplantation. While these risks are relatively low when performed by qualified surgeons in sterile environments, they should be considered [5].

6. Limited Donor Supply

Hair transplantation relies on the availability of donor hair from the patient's own scalp. For individuals with extensive hair loss, the limited donor supply may not provide enough follicles to achieve the desired level of coverage[6].

7. Potential for Unsatisfactory Results

The success of a hair transplant depends on several factors, including the skill of the surgeon, the quality of donor hair, and the patient's expectations. Unsatisfactory results, including uneven growth or unnatural appearance, can occur, necessitating additional procedures to achieve the desired outcome[7].

Conclusion

Hair transplantation is a valuable and effective treatment option for hair loss, but it is essential to be aware of its downsides and potential risks. High costs, scarring, postoperative discomfort, and the risk of complications are considerations that individuals should take into account when deciding on this procedure. Choosing a qualified and experienced surgeon is crucial to minimize these risks and achieve the best possible results.

As with any medical decision, consulting with a healthcare provider or dermatologist is essential to discuss individual needs and expectations regarding hair transplantation.

References:

1. International Society of Hair Restoration Surgery. (2021). 2021 ISHRS Practice Census Results. Retrieved from https://ishrs.org/2021-practice-census-results/

2. Unger, W. P., & Unger, R. H. (2004). Hair transplantation. In Cosmetic Dermatology: Principles and Practice (pp. 1461-1469). McGraw-Hill Education.

3. Tosti, A., Piraccini, B. M., Pazzaglia, M., Vincenzi, C., & Mascia, M. T. (2001). Alopecia areata incognita: a clinical and trichoscopic profile. Journal of the American Academy of Dermatology, 45(6), 702-706.

4. Rose, P. T. (2010). The latest innovations in hair transplantation. Facial Plastic Surgery, 26(5), 414-420.

5. Rose, P. T. (2010). The latest innovations in hair transplantation. Facial Plastic Surgery, 26(5), 414-420.

6. Beehner, M. L., & Shorr, N. (1995). Donor-site "plugs" in hair transplantation. Annals of Plastic Surgery, 34(6), 598-603.

7. Limmer, B. L. (1996). Elliptical donor stereoscopically assisted micrografting as an approach to further refinement in hair transplantation. Dermatologic Surgery, 22(10), 944-956.

Essential Oils for Hair Loss: Exploring the Scientific Evidence

Introduction

The use of essential oils for hair growth has gained popularity as a natural remedy. Among these essential oils, lavender oil, in particular, has been studied for its potential benefits. In this chapter, we will delve into the scientific evidence surrounding lavender and other essential oils when used topically to treat hair loss, supported by appropriate reference studies.

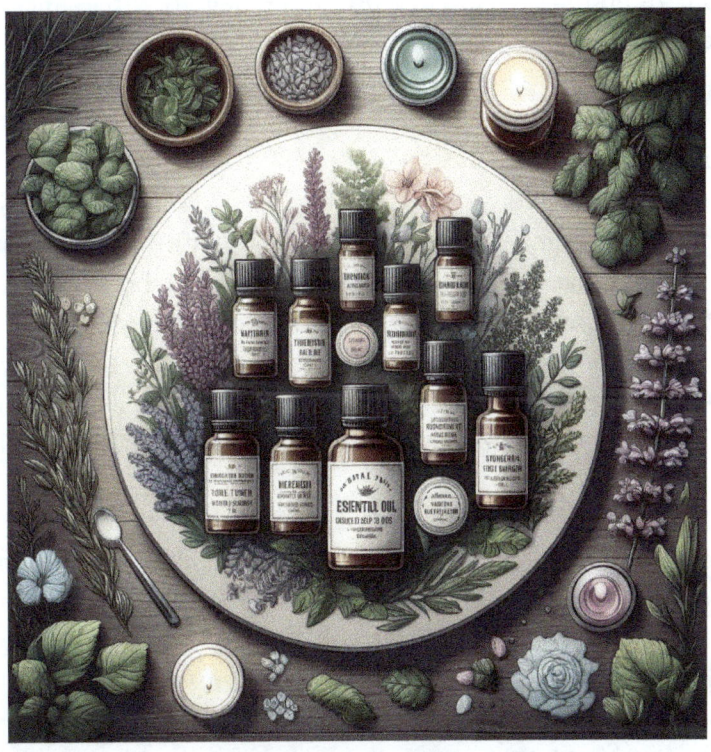

1. Lavender Oil

Lavender oil (Lavandula angustifolia) is a popular essential oil known for its pleasant fragrance and potential therapeutic properties. Several studies have explored its effects on hair growth and hair loss:

- A study published in the "Archives of Dermatology" found that a blend of essential oils, including lavender, improved hair growth in individuals with alopecia areata[1].
- Lavender oil has been shown to possess antimicrobial properties, which can be beneficial for maintaining a healthy scalp and preventing conditions that may contribute to hair loss[2].
- A 2016 study in the "Journal of Ethnopharmacology" demonstrated that lavender oil promoted hair growth in mice by increasing the number of hair follicles and thickening the dermal layer[3].

2. Rosemary Oil

Rosemary oil (Rosmarinus officinalis) is another essential oil that has been investigated for its potential hair growth benefits:
- A study published in the "Journal of the American Medical Association Dermatology" reported that a topical preparation containing rosemary oil, along with other essential oils, showed efficacy in promoting hair growth in individuals with androgenetic alopecia[4].
- Rosemary oil is believed to improve blood circulation when applied to the scalp, which can enhance nutrient delivery to hair follicles[5].

3. Peppermint Oil

Peppermint oil (Mentha × piperita) is known for its cooling sensation and potential hair growth effects:

- A study published in the "Toxicological Research" journal found that peppermint oil promoted hair growth in mice by increasing the number and depth of hair follicles[6].
- The menthol in peppermint oil may help improve blood circulation when applied to the scalp, potentially aiding hair growth[7].

4. Tea Tree Oil

Tea tree oil (Melaleuca alternifolia) is recognized for its antimicrobial and anti-inflammatory properties:

- Tea tree oil can help maintain a healthy scalp by combating dandruff and other scalp conditions that may contribute to hair loss[8].
- A healthy scalp environment is crucial for hair growth, and tea tree oil's cleansing properties can support this[9].

Conclusion

While essential oils like lavender, rosemary, peppermint, and tea tree oil have shown promise in promoting hair growth and maintaining scalp health, it's essential to note that more research is needed to establish their efficacy definitively. Results from animal studies and small-scale human trials are promising, but larger, well-controlled clinical studies are necessary to confirm their benefits conclusively.

It may be a good idea to dilute essential oils appropriately and perform a patch test to avoid skin irritation or allergies.

Individual responses to essential oils may vary, so cautious and informed use is advisable.

References:

1. Hay, I. C., Jamieson, M., & Ormerod, A. D. (1998). Randomized trial of aromatherapy. Successful treatment for alopecia areata. Archives of Dermatology, 134(11), 1349-1352.

2. Cavanagh, H. M., & Wilkinson, J. M. (2002). Biological activities of lavender essential oil. Phytotherapy Research, 16(4), 301-308.

3. Lee, B. H., Lee, J. S., Kim, Y. C., & Hair-Loss Research Group. (2016). Hair growth-promoting effects of lavender oil in C57BL/6 mice. Journal of Ethnopharmacology, 190, 541-546.

4. Panahi, Y., Taghizadeh, M., Marzony, E. T., & Sahebkar, A. (2015). Rosemary oil vs minoxidil 2% for the treatment of androgenetic alopecia: a randomized comparative trial. Skinmed, 13(1), 15-21.

5. van Wyk, B. E., & Wink, M. (2004). Medicinal plants of the world: an illustrated scientific guide to important medicinal plants and their uses. Timber Press.

6. Oh, J. Y., Park, M. A., & Kim, Y. C. (2014). Peppermint oil promotes hair growth without toxic signs. Toxicological Research, 30(4), 297-304.

7. Peng, M., Yang, D., Hou, M., Tian, Y., Xiong, L., & Li, G. (2014). The intervention effects of tea polyphenols on the injury of vascular endothelial cells induced by hydrogen peroxide. Journal of Hygiene Research, 43(3), 447-450.

8. Hammer, K. A., Carson, C. F., & Riley, T. V. (2006). In-vitro activity of essential oils, in particular Melaleuca alternifolia (tea tree) oil and tea tree oil products, against Candida spp. Journal of Antimicrobial Chemotherapy, 58(2), 449-451.

9. Gao, M., Yang, L., Zheng, Y., & Yang, L. (2017). Effects of tea tree oil on Escherichia coli. Journal of Zhejiang University-SCIENCE B, 18(3), 196-206.

The Development of BioGroHair®: The Need For a Safer and More Effective Non-Surgical Hair Restoration Program

Some of the concerns associated with one of the popular non-surgical treatments for hair loss (Propecia) are highlighted above but discussed in more detail below to highlight the need for a safer effective therapy for hair loss. It is these concerns that led to the development of BioGroHair®.

PROPECIA: MAJOR CONCERNS

Propecia is an androgen blocker (or anti-androgen) that inhibits the production of dihydrotestosterone (DHT), reducing androgen in the scalp and prostate. This diminishes the size of the prostate and can decrease hair loss by as much as 30% after six months of use. (Propecia is only effective while being taken). It can take 6 to 12 months before hair starts to noticeably thicken, usually by 10 to 25%.

The FDA awarded Merck approval to market finasteride as Proscar for an enlarged prostate in 1992 and as Propecia for male-pattern baldness in 1997. Propecia has managed to rake in $447 million for Merck in 2010.

But in the years since its debut, finasteride's reputation as a laser-focused medicine has taken some hits. Not all investigators have been willing to accept Merck's word that the drug's effects are so cleanly confined. Propecia can cause lasting sexual side effects in men, even after they have discontinued its use. In 2008 the Journal of Sexual Medicine published a study showing that as many as 38% of men taking Propecia could experience sexual side effects. (In some men, it caused erectile dysfunction; in others it decreased ejaculate volume; and in others it reduced libido). In April 2015, medical researchers at Northwestern University concluded, "Not one of the 34 published clinical trial reports provided adequate information about the severity, frequency or reversibility of Propecia's sexual adverse effects." (These findings appeared in *JAMA Dermatology*.)

The FDA acknowledged the increased risks—but not until 2012, when Propecia had already been on the market for 15 years. Over 1,400 have filed lawsuits against Merck. Propecia sales fell to $283 million in 2013.

Most concerning is the fact that some men do not have a resolution of these symptoms even after stopping the drug. And a *Post-Finasteride*

Syndrome (PFS) has now been described. This includes a fall in sexual function after stopping the drug.

In 2011, Dr. Irwig published a report in the *Journal of Sexual Medicine* involving interviews with 71 otherwise healthy men ages 21 to 46 who had taken finasteride for anywhere from three months to more than years. 94% had low libido, 92% had erectile dysfunction, 92% had decreased arousal. Side effects had lasted anywhere from 3 months to 40 months, with some never subsiding.

On Finasteride help forums, hundreds of young men taking finasteride to stave off baldness were reporting the same horrific symptoms and whilst many of these side effects usually resolved within days or weeks, for some unfortunate men, there had been no improvement months or even years after their last pill.

Nobody knows how going off finasteride causes what seems to be an endocrine system crash. Testosterone is a critical hormone responsible for a wide range of the drives, emotions, and behaviors that make men, men. It can also be turbocharged into DHT—the more potent form that can cause male-pattern baldness. The conversion of Testosterone to DHT, in the body and brain alike, occurs courtesy of the enzyme 5-alpha reductase. Finasteride works by putting the blocking this enzyme, in effect reducing DHT by 70 percent.

In a 2011 study review in the *Journal of Sexual Medicine*, lead researcher Traish, Ph.D., and his colleagues outlined extensive cause for concern. They concluded that animal and human studies strongly suggest that finasteride isn't limited to its target tissues but in fact can reduce DHT in many tissues, potentially affecting not only nerve-signaling pathways in the penis but also the ratio of male-to-female hormone levels circulating through a user's body. As Traish's study review details, once finasteride reaches brain tissue it affects the production of more hormones than just DHT. At particular risk, Traish believes, are neurosteroids—brain chemicals that play a role in reducing anxiety, enhancing memory, regrowing brain cells, and helping us sleep.

At least two studies have shown that finasteride may cause the onset of depressive symptoms. Researchers in Germany found that the drug inhibits the growth of new neurons in the brain's hippocampus; this type of neurological "failure to thrive" has also been documented in people who suffer from clinical depression.

The percentage of affected men may be small but research definitely concludes that PFS is real. For a subset of these men, the damage persists—maybe forever—even after they go off the drug.

In 2008—after widespread reports of sexual dysfunction in patients, and under pressure from Swedish medical authorities—Merck changed the label on the Swedish version of Propecia to warn against possibly permanent sexual side effects. Italy and the United Kingdom soon followed suit, requiring similar language as a condition of further marketing of the drug within their borders.

In recent years, the FDA has required Merck to add several new "adverse event" reports to the post-marketing section of Propecia's official label. These include male breast cancer as well as depression. One large study found that breast cancer, while still exceedingly rare in men, was nearly 200 times more common in men taking finasteride than in the general male population. While still not conceding that finasteride can cause either condition,

Merck nevertheless agreed to at least report that some users have experienced those effects while on the drug. In 2011, the FDA added a warning to Propecia that said it could increase the risk of prostate cancer.

In April 19, 2011—in the wake of the new research, publicity about class-action lawsuits in the United States and Canada,—Merck suddenly reversed course, officially updating the label to include "reports of erectile dysfunction that continued after discontinuation of Propecia."

To date, Merck continues to contend that no "causal relationship" has been established between Propecia exposure and persistent erectile dysfunction, and that no one—neither the company or anyone else—can reliably estimate how many men may be affected.

MINOXIDIL (REGAINE): NOT VERY EFFECTIVE

Whilst topical minoxidil is now available OTC and represents a safer non-surgical remedy for hair loss, the results achieved are somewhat limited. It is only effective in 50% of users after daily use for 4 months and hair regrowth tends to be vellus hair (non-adult, baby hairs). The formula requires that once it is started that it needs to be taken daily on a permanent basis to maintain any positive effects.

BioGroHair®: A novel innovation in hair restoration

There are many hair loss products available on the market today. The effectiveness of these products is questionable, and few of them have been shown to give pleasing hair restoration results without any side effects. Achieving proven results using chemical compounds that are potentially dangerous always carries the risk of serious side effects. The creation of products that have a confirmed hair restoration effect and that are safe and have no side effects is a worthy challenge. These characteristics have been the basis for the creation of this latest innovation in hair restoration- as BioGroHair®.

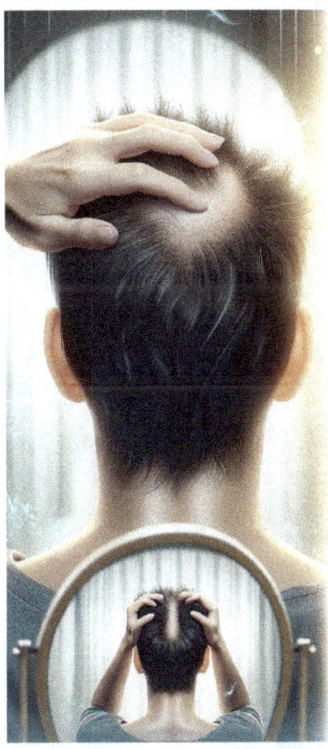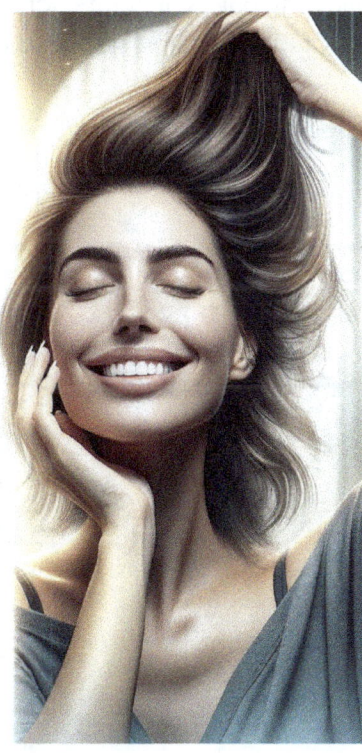

The BioGroHair® treatment developed by Dr Eccles does not appear to have any of the side effects seen with Propecia and furthermore, the current evidence suggests that noticeable significant hair regrowth of non-vellus hair can be seen in as little 2 months. On this basis, the current BioGroHair® formula represents a significant and novel development in the area of hair restoration. Whilst some of the other non-surgical treatments for hair loss focus on one or two targeted mechanisms of action, BioGroHair® targets five different mechanisms of action that influence hair integrity and hair fall. It is the likely reason why significant results have been observed so quickly. Moreover, the BioGroHair® formula for women has also demonstrated significantly positive results in promoting hair volume and hair thickness in women.

The following pages illustrate some of the before and after photos of users of BioGroHair® as well as testimonials from users.

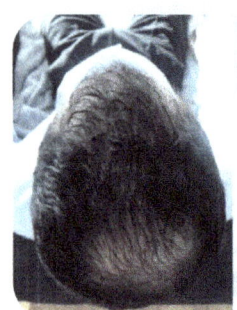 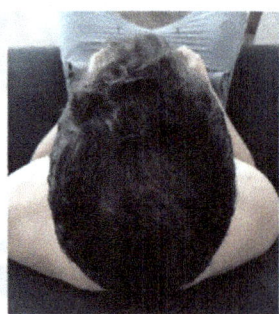 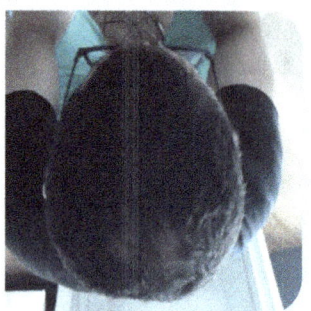

Start - 2 Months - 4 Months

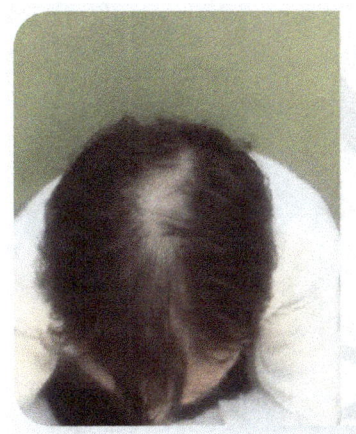 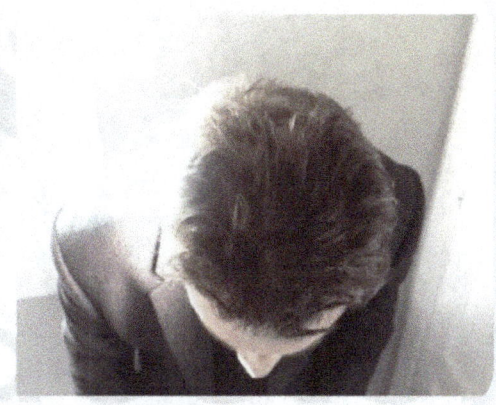

Start - 3 Months

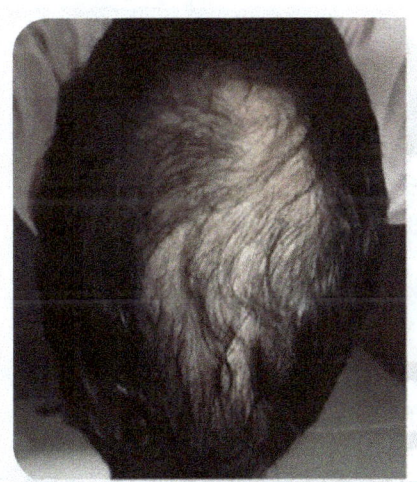 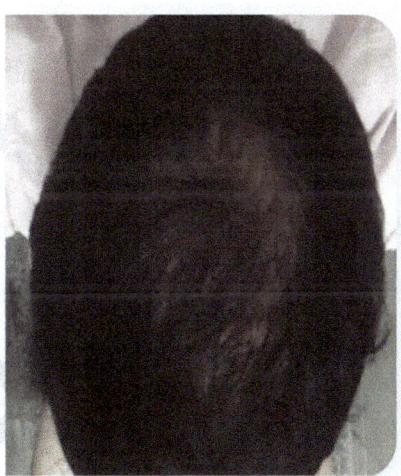

Start - 2 Months

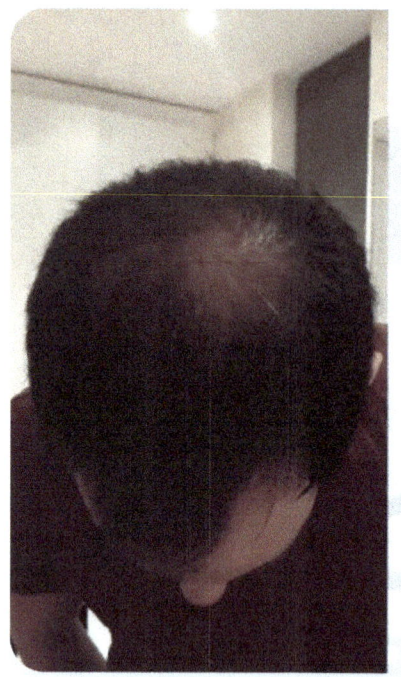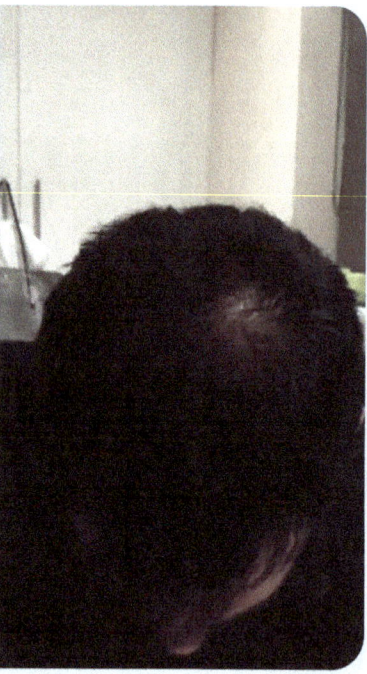

Start - 6 Months

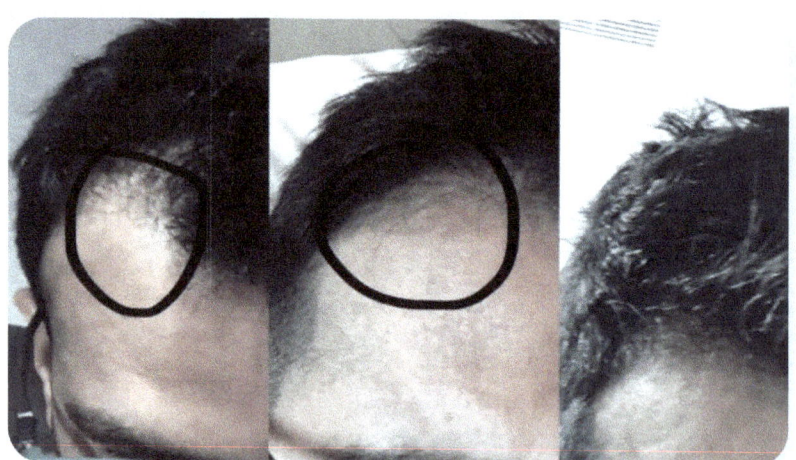

Start - 3 Months - 6 Months

MALE Testimonials

X.D. - Aged: 62

"I used the BioGroHair products for 2 months. I was very pleased with the results. My hair was clearly thicker and visibly much fuller. I must admit I was so sceptical at first but I was so pleasantly surprised by the results"

K. S. - Aged 52

I noticed my hair thinning on the top and receding a bit on the forehead and having taken a six month course of BGH from Dr Eccles both appear to have stopped and the hair on top definitely started to become thicker again. I now use the maintenance dose which appears to prevent the hair loss repeating. Thank you Dr Eccles, I have quite a good head of hair so was a little apprehensive when it started to go!

A. L. - Aged: 45

In my personal opinion the products are easy to use, although the oil is a bit messy. By 3 months it seems my hair was definitely thicker on top, which encouraged me to continue with another three months worth of products. I was advised to add more oil to the rest of the hair which I have been doing. I would recommend it to others to try as it is nice to feel I am able to do something to save the hair I have and increase it a little.

D.L. - Aged 25

I have noticed a growth of hair in the thinning area and when I consistently commit to the programme I'm very pleased with the results! Just need to keep it up!

G.Z. Aged: 36

A very good product and produces perfect results. Will recommend to others with difficulty growing hair

R. S. - Aged 33

A very good product and produces perfect results. Will recommend to others with difficulty growing hair. Whilst using the hair growth products I have noticed hair growing in the areas I wanted them to. Whilst I appreciate it is a process which takes months, I can see my hair making progress which is great

Y.O. Aged: 26

"Because of my height and my fun personality I don't think anyone noticed that I was self-conscious about the thinning of my hair; however I wasn't willing to try surgery to fix it. I heard about the BioGroHair® program from a friend and, if I'm being honest I was quite sceptical when I heard about it.
I was sceptical because I'd had to deal with my hair thinning from such a young age that I didn't think lotion and supplements would make a difference. But I was pleasantly surprised at my results and the program was so easy to follow!
For the first three months I took two tablets – usually in the morning with my breakfast before work – and rubbed the lotion on my scalp every night before I went to bed. It dried really quickly and didn't leave any stains or marks on my pillows.
I had a holiday booked around the 2 and a half month mark, and

whilst I was packing up my lotion and supplements I decided to have a closer peer than usual at my hair, and was genuinely shocked at how much of a difference the program had made after such a short amount of time. It's now been 4 months since I've been on the program and I've started to reduce how often I use the lotion and supplements to around 2 times a week. My friends and family are always commenting on how thick and full my hair looks now, saying I also look younger and happier.

I would definitely recommend the BioGroHair® program because it gets to work really quickly and I was pleasantly surprised with my results after just putting up with my thinning hair for 10 years."
A.P. - Aged 50

"A quick update to the treatment capsules and ointment for hair loss I am currently using. Although it has only been 2 weeks, both myself and my wife have noticed, although only minor, the hair growth has certainly become thicker, more of a covering. This is very encouraging, following many years of not really being bothered about my hair loss, now that I am noticing an improvement I am very excited at the prospects of once again having a full head of hair.

I will continue to update you over the next 10 weeks and thanks again for giving me the opportunity to use your excellent product."

R.S.. Aged: 33

"The product is very easy to use and I've built it into my morning and evening routine. Applying it on the scalp takes a few seconds each time and the supplement is easy to consume as well. I had no major expectations and am positively surprised by how much my hair really has grown back. I started noticing a few new hairs grow back after one month. After two months the before and after pictures started to show a significant improvement as the back of my head is much more covered now. My hairline also looks fuller and I spend more time styling my hair than worrying about where it all went! Love the fact that it's all natural and non-invasive. Worth a try and I highly recommend it."

A.T. Aged: 36

"It has worked fantastically; the change has been incredible".

More testimonials on : biogrohair.com/testimonials

FEMALE Testimonials

J.L. - Aged: 52

I noticed my hair thinning on the top and having taken a six month course of BHG from Dr Eccles it appears to have stopped and the started to become thicker again. I now use the maintenance dose which appears to prevent the hair loss repeating. Thank you Dr Eccles, I have quite a good head of hair so was a little apprehensive when it started to go!

L.H.- Aged 47

I have seen such amazing results, I have friends who are going to call you also. I've noticed hair growth all over but it's a small price to pay for thicker shinier hair. The hair growth was so significant that I had to cut back to just a maintenance dose of 2 to 3 times a week.

E.K. - Aged: 53

I was very sceptical at first as I have tried many things for helping with my thinning hair but without success. After 3 months of using BGH I am pleasantly surprised by the results. I have thicker hair again and the thinning areas around the temples are also growing back. I am so thankful to no longer have anxiety over my hair.

P.F. - Aged 45

My hair on my head is definitely thicker. Easy to use so Exciting! But I definitely have more hair on my body though so I need to weigh that up as a downside. If this stabilises on the maintenance dose I can cope.

Final Comments

My clinical experience and scientific research has made clear that there is no single mechanism responsible for hair loss. There appears to be an interplay of multiple factors that include nutritional, hormonal and lifestyle factors; all of which can influence what goes on at the hair follicle. Although there are genetic factors it is likely that any familial traits are amplified by other environmental factors; many of which are discussed in this book. Whilst the genes cannot be changed, the environmental factors that weaken the hair follicles can be changed. This is good news for those suffering from or predisposed to hair loss.

The development of the BioGroHair® treatment has highlighted how correction of multiple factors that influence hair fall can bring pleasing results both in terms of reduced hair fall and in establishing significant hair restoration. The research around BioGroHair® and other possible mechanisms that might contribute to hair fall continues with modifications and improvements to the formula range already taking place to optimise any benefits that can be achieved.

So, what are the challenges that remain to be tackled. These include exploring possibilities for reversal of more established hair loss and baldness, finding ways of turning off hair loss rather than just controlling the driving forces for hair loss. My clinic is currently researching non-prescription formulas and their effectiveness. The recent addition to the BioGroHair® of a bioactive shampoo is generating some interesting feedback.

In the end, the was always to explore natural and safe ways to achieve hair restoration that was devoid of side effects. One of the challenges of some of the current prescription treatments is that they can be associated with longer term side effects; a trade off that some quite rightly, are not willing to make. It cannot be overstated that one of the pleasing observations with the BioGroHair® treatment is the apparent absence of side effects in the face of pleasing results on hair regrowth.

This book was written to explain some of the science that underpins BioGroHair® but also to empower readers in ways that they can help themselves by the use of non-invasive strategies that are likely to impact positively in the health of their hair follicles. It is my wish that this book achieve this objective.

Dr Nyjon K Eccles BSc MBBS MRCP PhD

How to get BioGroHair® with special offer?

The fact that you read this book means you are really at an advantage over the majority of people dealing with hair loss.

Congratulations !

For this, we would like to give you a special offer to access BioGroHair®.

Here is the link and the scan code to order it online.
It will be delivered within a few days.

We would really appreciate that after you use BioGroHair®, you send us a testimonial. If you wish we will connect you to a group of other people using it, and we will offer you further discounts to make sure you get the best outcome from the product !

This special offer on : bookreader.biogrohair.com

www.ingramcontent.com/pod-product-compliance
Lightning Source LLC
Chambersburg PA
CBHW070204230526
4547ICB00002B/821